Flexible Dieting: Crush Those Cravings, Eat What You Want and Still Lose Weight

Jennifer Cox

Author's Note

I really want to thank you for downloading this book and wish you the best of success in implementing these strategies. I wanted to talk about my story – not to be boastful – but to serve as motivation to my readers :)

From a young age my diet consisted of junk food several times a week and anything that I could microwave. I often would hit the drive through 5 times a week. This coupled with little to no exercise meant that I ballooned through my teenage years to eventually **400 pounds**.

It all came one fateful day, when looking at pictures, I couldn't believe what I was seeing. I saw myself as the obese, unhealthy and unattractive woman I was. I went through the infamous cycle of acceptance. At first it was denial, "I'm not THAT big, am I?", "The camera adds 10 (more like 100) pounds" were some of the justifications I used. I eventually slowly began to slide into depression and this lasted several months. I began popping pills to help improve my mood, despite knowing what needed to be done. I eventually reached a stage where I knew I needed to change.

I began exercising, eating right and mixing with the right people. I worked hard and at times it was torture. I began to learn about correct food choices and how bad the food was that I was previously eating. As the pounds started coming off I increased my activity rate and continued with my (flexible) diet. I was able to bring my weight down to **160 pounds**.

My journey was a long and arduous one, and one which demanded greater mental strength than physical. I have written this book in the hope of informing people who are in the same position I was a few years ago.

Before you go any further, I must stress, though the diet plan is vital, you won't follow through on it without the acceptance of your mind. For this reason, I suggest you read: Weight Loss Motivation Hacks – which were some techniques I used to rewire my mind to help me reach my goals. It is available on the Amazon and CreateSpace store.

I hope this book is informative and helps you in achieving the body you have always dreamed of.

You can do it!

Table of Contents

Author's Note

Table of Contents

Chapter 1 – Don't Suffer Any Longer
What is Dieting?
Why Dieting Doesn't Have to Be a Horrible Experience
Why You Should Stop Restricting Yourself
The Good Food/Bad Food Myth

Chapter 2 – Flexible Dieting 101
What is Flexible Dieting?
Can I Really Eat Anything I Want?
My Fiber Needs
The Benefits of Flexible Dieting

Chapter 3 – Calorie Counting is King
What is a Calorie?
How Many Calories Do I Need?
Does it Matter How Many Protein, Carbohydrates or Fats I Consume?
How Can I Track My Calories?
How Many Times a Day Should I Eat?
Meal Timing
I'm Ready to Get Started!
Tips and Tricks to Succeed in Your Goals

Chapter 4 – Examples of Full Days of Eating
Day 1 – McDonalds
Day 2 – Burger King
Day 3 – McDonalds, KFC and Domino's
Tips
Additional Suggested Meals

Chapter 5 – Supplementation
Do I Need Supplements for Weight Loss?
Which Types of Supplements Could be Beneficial for Me?
Thermogenics
Stimulant-free Weight Loss Supplements
Carb Blockers

Fat Blockers
Appetite Suppressants
Cortisol Blockers
Vitamin D Supplementations
Supplements for Each Gender
Supplements by their Active Ingredient
Yohimbine
Calcium
African Mango Extract
Bitter Orange
Capsaicin
Chromium Picolinate
Diatomaceous Earth
Green Tea Extract
Omega 3 Fatty Acid
Caffeine

Conclusion

Chapter 1 – Don't Suffer Any Longer

What is Dieting?

Each individual has their own lifestyle, metabolism and work. It is the intensity of the work which determines the quantity and the nature of food that a particular individual requires, in order to survive. This food is converted into energy (scientifically speaking, it yields Adenosine Tri-phosphate or ATP), which is used up in daily activities.

Recent trends in technology have forced the human race to work less (physically speaking) and eat more. The quantity has not suffered major changes, but the quality of food has. Can you imagine how much simpler food from the forties or fifties was compared to the present day? The calorie intake has increased majorly because of the complexity and the fat content of the food. The decreased levels of physical activity have made it difficult to burn those calories. Where do the extra calories go? They get stored in the body in the form of fats for the times when food is not available.

Dieting is a common measure sought to deprive the body from food (ATP), which will help it shed those extra pounds. The fat must melt to compensate for the shortage in energy. A million evil alterations have crept into this simple concept in an attempt to find shortcuts for those who are lazy or too busy to make these efforts. Some alterations that have crept in this concept cause more harm than good.

Through my journey, I have been able to dig through the layers upon layers of myths to unleash the true meaning of dieting. Dieting is simply a synonym to eating right. Eating anything you want, but *the correct amount*. This method has allowed me to shed all my extra baggage and still maintain my sanity by eating my favorite foods. It's possible and I am testament to it.

Why Dieting Doesn't Have to Be a Horrible Experience

A huge misconception with dieting is that it is all fruits, vegetables and lean meats (*Yuck!*). But with flexible dieting this is not the full story. Wouldn't it be awesome to eat without compromising on your taste buds and cravings? Flexible dieting allows you to do that.

As we discussed, each person has their own lifestyle, metabolism and work. This means each of us has a certain amount of energy or calories (see Chapter 3) that we need to consume in order to lose, gain or maintain weight. Flexible dieting teaches that you can eat *whatever* you wish, as long as it is within the parameters of your daily caloric goal. I will show you (Chapter 4) how I have eaten at all of my favorite fast-food joints and stayed within my calorie goal.

Why You Should Stop Restricting Yourself

I can guarantee you've been through this: you look in the mirror and don't see what you like. Your confidence takes a huge hit and you find it difficult to be approach other men/women. The outcome is usually gnawing on raw fruits or vegetables, halfheartedly in the hope that this will help us achieve our dream body. However, is this really an option? Of course, you will lose weight at once. Nevertheless, crash dieting has its own set of repercussions. In fact, it has more repercussions than benefits.

When you restrict yourself from consuming the food item of your choice, your body tends to eat up all the reserves of glycogen in the liver and then proceed towards muscle and finally, on to fats. Thus, you do lose weight drastically but it is of no use, since you have begun losing muscles and it is slowly beginning to turn into a hollow shell.

Finally, if you restrict all the food you like, then it is likely that you will give it up sooner than later. Nobody likes to compromise on food and if you follow a restrictive diet, you will succumb to temptations, much before you realize it. Flexible dieting is more effective than the latter, when it comes to reaching your goal. The body eventually gets tired on compromising and before you know it, you are indulging in much more food than you were eating even before your diet!

The Good Food/Bad Food Myth

Food is food. Food cannot be good or bad. The body needs every food group: fats, proteins and carbohydrates. Of course, the portion size acts as the boundaries for each food group (see later). The body has its own mechanism and you must strictly obey certain rules to remain fit and healthy. Portion sizes are simply one of them. For example, an average male must consume 2640 calories with 300g of carbohydrates, 150-200 g of protein and 40 – 70g of fats. If you consume either carbohydrates or fats in excess amount, the body will retain it and this will lead to weight gain.

It is a common misconception that weight loss journey has to be a painstakingly difficult task to conquer for the dieter. However, this as mentioned before, is a wrong concept. Dieting has been wrongly labeled as depriving yourself of all the delicious food and adapting yourself to a strenuous lifestyle.

What I aim to inform you here is that if you are unhappy with your diet right now, you are certainly not doing it the **right way**. It is high time that you give up on all that makes you unhappy and you start eating at your own wishes and still not gain weight, but of course, you must be cautious of the calorie count.

Good or bad food items are a myth. We agree that a few nutrient groups can remain stored in the body, but even they are important, up to certain extent. Therefore, to remain at the peak of your health, you must consume everything but at the same time, you must know your limits as well. Biding by these limits will not only nourish your body but shall also help you from falling prey to numerous diseases.

Chapter 2 – Flexible Dieting 101

What is Flexible Dieting?

Flexible dieting is a growing trend in the sector of fitness, dieting and healthy eating. Otherwise known as "If it Fits Your Macros or IIFYM", it emphasizes on how you need to make adjustments with macronutrients, namely, carbohydrates, fats and proteins in your diet.

Most often than not, we are overpowered by our cravings when on a diet. This diet plan plans a composition goal for the dieter. Therefore, flexible dieters like to believe that food can be neither good nor bad (Chapter 1); that weight cannot be lost by skipping or adding meals but you sure can work miracles with the combination of ratios of food groups. It believes in the universal fact that the body and the metabolism does not infer healthy and unhealthy, it simply breaks down the food to release energy.

Can I *Really* Eat Anything I Want?

The short answer is a resounding YES! Flexible dieting suggests that you can eat a McGrilled Burger or tuna with brown rice (boring) and the same amount of macronutrients shall reach your body, 25g protein, 15g fat and 33g carbohydrates. This is because of the same nature of the macronutrients. Clearly, it does not matter what goes into your body unless and until you meet your calorie goals.

My Fiber Needs

Flexible dieting allows users to eat what they want, provided they stay in their limits. The truth is that health has been redefined with flexible eating. According to flexible dieting, a follower must be eating fourteen grams of fiber per thousand calories. For example, if you consume an average of three thousand calories, then you must consume 3 x 14= 52 grams of fiber. When you increase your fiber intake, you will fulfill most of your micro nutrition needs and keep your cholesterol levels in check. A single shot hitting multiple targets.

The Benefits of Flexible Dieting

Effective

When you are not consuming more calories than you need, you are maintaining a balance between the energy you utilize with the food you eat. With regular meals and snacks, you can effectively maintain a constant supply of energy. Thus, flexible dieting is effective in a number of situations be it gaining, maintaining and losing weight.

Flexible (*duh!*)

It's in the name, you don't have to be conscious of the health benefits of everything single thing you put in your mouth. Instead, you can have variety in your diet components from time to time. When you do so, you are giving your taste buds the opportunity to relish good food but since you are maintaining a macro ratio, you need not worry about gaining weight.

Sustainable

It helps to kill the restrictive dieting and bingeing cycle. Experts say how single days of bingeing throughout the week can disrupt the cycle. Thus, with flexible dieting, you can effectively control your urges. It is best to maintain a regular flow instead of incorporating small changes into your diet from time to time.

Chapter 3 – Calorie Counting is King

What is a Calorie?

A calorie is a scientific unit of measurement of energy. If you scan the internet or the encyclopedia (if you're old school that is!) it would provide the usual definition of how much energy you would need to raise the temperature of one gram of water by one degree Celsius. However, when we refer to dieting, we say that a particular food item bears a certain amount of calories. What we mean is that when that food item is completely digested by the human body, it releases that many calories of energy. This energy, thus generated is used to perform work. The calories that exceeds the amount you need is stored as fats leading to weight gain. Our aim here is to lose those excess fats (in other words, utilize the fat and digest it.) and become fit.

How Many Calories Do I Need?

Each one of us has a different lifestyle. Our levels of activities, eating patterns and body metabolism define our ideal calories intake on a daily basis. Thus, there is no single "works for all policy" in the case of calorie intake. To figure out the amount of calories you need, you need the basic information about your body, including age, height, weight and Body Mass Index (BMI). Body Mass Index, as the name suggests, is the ratio between the weight and the muscle content (since muscle can also burn calories.)

Regulating your daily activity level as well as your calorie intake is the sole means of maintain, losing and gaining weight. To figure out your appropriate action that you must adapt, you must know your ideal calorie intake. It can be easily calculated using your computer! Use: http://bit.ly/howmanycaloriesshouldieat

Does it Matter How Many Protein, Carbohydrates or Fats I Consume?

A single gram of carbohydrates and proteins each contain four calories each, whereas a gram of fats contains nine calories. Irrespective of the quality of the food, as long as you consume only the amount of calories that you need, you will be just fine. So let's say hypothetically, you want to consume 360 calories for one of your meals/snacks. You can theoretically consume 40g of fat in the form of olive oil (though I'm not sure why you would!).

How Can I Track My Calories?

In this age where smart phones are the craze, you should definitely not be asking this question! Had it been the eighties or the nineties, you would have to seek appointment from the nutritionist, run to them a few times and then have the diet chart with us.

However, in recent times where drastic changes can be made at the gesture of a fingertip, you can select an app which will keep track of your calorie intake for you. Just make sure to make an entry every time you snack or eat, something including its portion size. I

use an app called MyFitnessPal, check it out:
https://www.myfitnesspal.com/

How Many Times a Day Should I Eat?

The usual concept of three meals everyday is outdated. Flexible dieting allows you to eat as many times as you want. You can eat two times a day or eight times a day, it's your call! However, you need to ensure that you count the calories while eating. So long as the amount of calories stays the same, it does not matter if you eat twice a day or eight times, a day! This is the beauty of flexible dieting. It not only gives you the flexibility, but also allows you to take charge of what you are going to eat and what you are going to avoid. It helps you to remain sane and follow this diet as a lifestyle, instead of a diet!

Meal Timing

When should you have your breakfast/lunch/dinner? It is not possible to assign a particular time for each meal. You cannot always have lunch, for example, exactly at 1 o' clock. There can be a lot of commitments before you sit down to eat. At the same time, you cannot simply eat as and when you feel like.

First and foremost, never skip your breakfast. Let us classify people into two types; those who exercise in morning and those who do not. Make sure to eat your breakfast within an hour after you wake up, if you do not exercise in the morning. This will help you keep your blood sugar level regulated and also helps to avoid a high carbohydrate meal out of hunger, later during the day. If you are aiming at weight loss, have your breakfast immediately after exercising. There are no concrete proofs but, there are small studies performed by Journal of Physiology which demonstrate that is the best time.

If you are not able to consume your breakfast as per above, make sure to consume it before 10 am. It is the golden rule of breakfast. Your lunch time depends on various factors including your work schedule. It is better to leave a gap of 4-5 hours between your breakfast and lunch.

If you have a 9-5 job, make sure to have your dinner before 7. Generally, a person with a normal job schedule would not be burning a lot of calories after 7 in the evening. Thus, a high carbohydrate filled meal after 7 can increase sugar levels in your body. If you have an active evening life, consume dinner 3-4 hours, before your bed time.

I'm Ready to Get Started!

Flexible dieting requires setting effective goals. The goal setting is a critical step in the process. If you are not well informed, things could go horribly wrong. Following is a brief few points which will help you get started.

Evaluate your present diet to gather information about your daily caloric intake

From free tools available online to various articles and guides which talk extensively of calculating your macros, you have large number of options. All that you must do is utilize the information available.

Get Yourself a Food Scale

A food scale contains accurate details about the nutritional components of each of the food items. Even though the food packaging contains ample information about the nutrient contents, a food scale comes handy especially if you are the extra cautious kinds.

Track Your Progress

As explained before, a number of apps are available for tracking and measuring your calorie intake. I recommend this app called MyFitnessPal available for Mac, Windows and Android, it is the world's largest nutritional database.

Tips and Tricks to Succeed in Your Goals

1. Plan so that you do not have to spend a lot of time thinking what you want to eat. Planning your meals beforehand will also help you to figure out ways you can indulge. So what are you waiting for?

2. Most of us tend to lose interest in our diets because the food items we consume tend to make it boring. So in order to please your taste buds and not let the extra calories pile up, you must include some items of your choice in the diet (Chapter 4). You must keep a keen eye on the calorie count at the same time as well.

3. It is advisable to calculate the amount of protein you're going to eat. At least 20g of protein are needed by the body to begin synthesizing muscle protein. Subsequent minor drops can be supplemented in subsequent meals or protein supplementation.

4. Balanced meals are the key to success in the sphere of fitness. The Glycaemic Index (GI) tends to go down as you include more proteins, fats, fibre, and consuming carbohydrates. Thus, with more protein and fibre, you need not worry about the imbalance caused to GI levels.

5. Even though flexible dieting does not believe in the conventional concept of good food and bad food, you must understand that fresh fruits and vegetables are a great source of fibre and micronutrients, which play a key role in the nourishment of the body and the conductance of various vital physiological processes. So make sure you include these when eating.

6. For your diet to be flexible and in order to avoid hitting those minor bumps, it is best that you leave some room for the flexibility. Otherwise, an occasional change of plans for dinner, lunch or brunches could leave you falling off your plans.

Chapter 4 – Examples of Full Days of Eating

Now that we have talked about how to track calories, how to spread them over a day and how much to consume, this chapter will talk in detail about examples of full days of eating.

These are the exact meals I have eaten on numerous occasions while losing over 200 lbs. IT IS POSSIBLE! This diet plan consists of 2500 to 3000 calories, per day. This is not a constant value. This calorie limit depends on various factors as you would have learnt in Chapter 3.

Day 1 – McDonalds

Total macronutrients for the day: 102g protein, 229g of carbohydrates and 48g of fat. Total calories: (102x4) +(229x4) +(48x9) = 1756 calories

Breakfast:

- Egg Omelet with White Bread (23g of protein, 46g of carbohydrates and 16g of fats)
- Orange (15-20g of fiber and 30g of carbohydrates)

Lunch:

- McGrilled Chicken Burger (25g of protein, 33g of carbohydrate and 15g of fat)
- Fresh Orange Juice (5 grams of fiber and 30 grams of carbohydrates)

Snack:

- Granola Bar and Peanut Butter Smoothie (27g of protein, 60g of carbohydrates, 15g of fat and 5g of fiber)

Dinner:

- Tuna Salad with Large Serving of Broccoli (27g of protein, 25g of carbohydrates and 4g of fat and 6.6g of fiber)

Day 2 – Burger King

Total macronutrients for the day: 49g of protein, 103g of carbohydrates and 20.2g of fat. Total calories: (49x4) +(103x4) +(20.2x9) = 800 calories.

Breakfast:

- Fruit 'n Yogurt Parfair (11g of carbohydrates, 5g of fat and 3g of fiber)
- Fruit Smoothie (15g of carbohydrates and 25-35g of fiber)

Lunch:

- Beef Steak with Potato, Sweet Potato and Broccoli (35g of protein, 30g of carbohydrates, 4.2g of fat and 3g of fiber)

Snack:

- Oat Smoothie and Fruit Salad (15g of carbohydrates, 2g of fat and 10g of fiber)

Dinner:

- Burger King Hamburger (14g of protein, 32g of carbohydrates, 9g of fat and 1g of fiber)

Day 3 – McDonalds, KFC and Domino's

Total macronutrients for the day: 113g of protein, 120g of carbohydrates and 72g of fat. Total calories: (113x4) +(120x4) +(72x9) = 1600 calories.

Breakfast:

- Egg McMuffin (18g of protein, 30g of carbohydrates and 12g of fat)
- Sausage Burrito (12g of protein, 26g of carbohydrates and 16g of fat)

Lunch:

- BBQ Sandwich KFC (24g of protein, 47g of carbohydrates, 3.5g of fat and 3g of fiber)

Snack:

- Apple Smoothie with Almond Milk (32g of protein, 20g of carbohydrates, 10g of fat and 5g of fiber)
- Dried Apricots (7g of protein, 3g of fat and 5g of fiber)

Dinner: Chicken Pizza (Domino's) (20g of protein, 50g of carbohydrates, 30g of fat and 4g of fiber)

Tips

This meals can be modified, as per your requirements. You need to keep a few tips in mind, before modifying or creating a diet plan:

1. The macro levels are not accurate. Sugar comes in different names and most of the times companies provide carbohydrate gained from just sugar. Read the label in detail.

2. Just because my meals have some fast food item on each day, this does not mean that you can eat in a fast food restaurant everyday and stay *healthy*. This diet shows how to incorporate your tasty choices, while maintaining a healthy diet.

3. You can also add an extra snack between breakfast and lunch. It is better to add another meal with nutrient filled food items than to just grab some snacks to fill your appetite or stay hungry and shovel your lunch.

Additional Suggested Meals

1. Wendy's grilled chicken with orange juice or ice tea (medium cup) (480 calories with 7g of fat and 50g of carbohydrate)

2. Fresco beef tacos (2) from Taco bell with Mexican rice (17g of fat, 45g of carbohydrate amounting to 470 calories)

3. Beef sub from Subway with Italian dressing and ice tea (8g of fat, 38g of carbohydrate and 14g of protein).

4. Honey bourbon chicken with chili cup from Quiznos (11.5g of fat, 46g of carbohydrate and 15g of protein)

5. Thin pizza with diet coke from Pizza hut accounts for 12 g of fat, 32g of carbohydrate and 19g of protein).

This is flexible dieting. You are free to change your meals as you wish, unless you are going beyond limits of macros. Make a schedule with healthy food and foods you love to eat. Create a balanced diet and stick to it. It might not be easy in the beginning. No matter how flexible your diet may be, you will be resistant to changes. It is human nature. Do not forgo dieting the moment you think you are not able to keep up with your plan. Take one step at a time.

Chapter 5 – Supplementation

Supplements are exactly that – they are there to supplement your diet and exercise plan. The majority of people who follow a diet take supplements. Dietary supplements contain herbal products, enzymes, vitamins, minerals, amino acids and other products. These supplements can be consumed via drinks, powder, bars, pills and various other forms.

Do I Need Supplements for Weight Loss?

The short answer is no; but they can help. I would advise that you consult your physician before embarking on any diet changes and/or taking weight loss supplements.

Firstly, it is important to make the distinction between drugs/medicines and supplements. Drugs are chemicals which are designed to have a specific therapeutic effect. Supplements are similar, with less side effects. Both are sometimes derived from natural sources. For example, aspirin is made from the bark tree. Drugs generally have a greater side effect profile than supplements derived by natural means.

Supplements boost one factor in your body which would aid weight loss, when combined with exercise and diet. People usually recommend starting the dieting process without supplements. If you think that you are not reducing considerable amount of weight even after three months of exercise and diet, you can start taking supplements – though this should be with caution. Look at your calorie intake and other factors, why haven't you lost weight after three months if you have followed a good diet? Instead of opting for supplements immediately, you should try to fix any leakages, in your diet, if any!

Which Types of Supplements Could be Beneficial for Me?

There are a lot of supplements which are focused on weight loss. The characteristics of supplements depend on its main active ingredient. Each supplement works in a different way in our body. This section will discuss the different types of fat loss supplements available on the market, how they work and if they would it be beneficial for you.

Thermogenics

As the name indicates, this supplement increases body temperature and helps to burn more calories. This is done by the first main ingredient, Caffeine. Yes, caffeine comes from coffee. But, no matter how many cups of coffee you consume every day, caffeine in your coffee will not perform this action. The next main ingredient is Yohimbine. This ingredient helps in dissolving fats from underlying fat cells. This type of supplement is for those who are not able to let go of those last few pounds from belly, thigh or any other part of body.

Stimulant-free Weight Loss Supplements

Most weight loss supplements have any one or more stimulants which increase activeness and alertness of subject. This stimulation helps in two ways. It helps subject to be active and thus, a lot of calories are burned. It also increases alertness and thus, people do not feel tired or need to consume a lot of food.

Common stimulants in supplements are caffeine, ephedra and others. Ephedra and many other stimulants are banned in a few countries. Moreover, many people are allergic to these stimulants. Common side effects are red face, agitation, jitters and others. If you have any such side effects while using any supplement, you can shift to stimulant-free supplement or contact your physician.

Carb Blockers

Carb blockers or carbohydrate blockers do exactly what their name indicates. It prevents the body from digesting and absorbing carbohydrates. Certain enzymes are produced by the body, to digest carbohydrates. This supplement reduces enzyme production and thus, carbohydrates you consume are not digested and are expelled from body. Thus, even if you consume limited amount of carbs, this supplement would reduce its storage. This type of supplement helps those who cheat a lot in their dieting. Even if you cheat for a day or two in a week, this supplement would expel carbohydrates from your body.

Fat Blockers

Fat blockers are very similar to carbohydrate blockers. The main ingredient in both supplements is chitosan. This ingredient is a fat absorbent. It absorbs fat from digestive tract. Chitosan cannot be digested by the human body and thus, chitosan along with fat would be expelled from body. Thus, you can lose weight without fat-free eating.

Chitosan removes approximately 10 calories from a person per day. The only disadvantage is that all minerals and vitamins which are soluble in fat also get expelled from body. Therefore, you might experience vitamin or mineral deficiency.

Appetite Suppressants

This is the most common weight loss supplement which a lot of people use – they are often prescribed by a physician. Before going in depth about this supplement, let us learn about our digestive mechanism. When the body is in need of energy, the body send signals in the form of brain chemicals or hormones which makes you feel hungry. After you are full, the body again creates brain signals, indicating you to stop eating as you are full.

The main aim of this supplement is to mimic brain signals which indicate that you are full. Thus, you will feel full, even when you are not. This would reduce your hunger and thereby, you would be consuming less. Consuming less amount of food is the first rule of dieting.

This type of supplement is preferred by medical professionals for those who are obese and for those who have eating problem or stress eating. There are mixed reviews about this product.

Cortisol Blockers

Let us talk about stress eating briefly. Those who have a stress eating problem tend to eat a lot (usually food rich in sugar) when they are stressed. For these people, most of the supplements mentioned above would not be effective.

Even if the subject follows a strict diet, when they are stressed, they become hungry and eat a lot. When a person is stressed, the body releases cortisol hormone. This is also called as stress hormone. Cortisol increases blood sugar, blood pressure and reduces strength of immunity. When cortisol is released in the body, it increases appetite. Moreover, deposited fat in body also releases signals which further increase appetite. When a person is stressed, these two factors act upon them and make them eat as much as possible.

Cortisol blockers helps in reducing stress hormone, thereby reducing all above mentioned scenarios. Much like appetite suppressants – cortisol blockers are often prescribed by physicians.

Vitamin D Supplementations

Vitamin D increases insulin sensitivity in the body. If your body is more sensitive, you tend to need lesser amount of calories and calories you do consume are less likely to end up as fat cells. Vitamin D deficiency reduces secretion of leptin, a hormone which indicates to the brain that body is full.

There is a considerable difference between this supplement and that of an appetite suppressor. Appetite suppressors mimics signals and makes you feel full even when you are not. Vitamin D pills would just increase effectiveness of production of leptin. Thus, when you are full, the body would immediately release leptin without any delay.

The second difference is that appetite suppressor works with the nervous system which may have some side effects. However, vitamin D pills do not alter brain signals and are thus safer to consume.

Supplements for Each Gender

Women and men do not have the same metabolic rate. Men are more potent with high stimulant products. They can handle products with more caffeine. Moreover, since men have better metabolism rate, supplements that increase metabolism rate are not usually very effective.

Women should use products that deal with stress, hormones, appetite and metabolism. Men should use products which deal with fat burning and removal of underlying fat cells.

Supplements by their Active Ingredient

The active ingredient in a supplement determines its characteristics. If you are not sure which type of supplement to use, you can use this section to choose supplements with the desirable active ingredient. There are a few constant ingredients, which are found in almost all supplements.

Yohimbine

This element helps in removing underlying fat cells. These cells are found in the lower abdomen, thigh and hip areas. Thus, those who want to shed those few pounds from the stomach or leg to regain their beautiful figure should use supplements with this element.

Calcium

Calcium helps in aiding vitamin D to remove fat (see Vitamin D Supplementation). When fat cell absorbs calcium, it tends to release fat. Moreover, when you consume calcium, fat gets attached to GI tract and this helps in promoting weight loss. This ingredient is essential for those who are consuming vitamin D pills for weight loss.

African Mango Extract

This ingredient helps in increasing the rate of metabolism. It is better to avoid this ingredient, unless you know that the product is of a high quality. It is one of many natural products which help in weight loss. African mango is not the common mango which you get in the grocery store. This fruit just resembles mango in its structure.

Bitter Orange

This ingredient is for those who want to reduce their hunger. It is a citrus fruit and has no harmful stimulant in it. There are no side effects of bitter orange extract and thus, can be used by everyone.

Capsaicin

Consuming a lot of spicy food will increase the rate of metabolism. This helps in weight loss. Moreover, spicy food would help you suppress your appetite.

Capsaicin is the element in all spicy food like chilly, pepper and others that make it hot.

Capsaicin extract is not spicy. It is just an extract from red pepper. This helps in reducing weight and also to avoid gaining weight back after weight loss. This supplement should be used by those who have achieved their target in weight loss and want to stick to their new weight without gaining it back.

Chromium Picolinate

This chemical reduces craving and stabilizes sugar levels. Thus, it will help you have more energy throughout the day, without relying on snacks and other refreshment. With less cravings, you can reduce cheating and also be more satisfied with your new diet. This chemical does not aid in weight loss. It just removes craving and thus, has to be combined with other weight loss factors like diet, exercise and supplements.

Diatomaceous Earth

This is powdered algae. This powder helps in detoxing your body and thereby, reducing weight with little effort from your end. There are no side effects and it helps in developing healthy hair, nail and gums. It also helps in reducing cholesterol and blood pressure. All you need to make sure is that it is a food grade product. There are a lot of fake products on the market and I would suggest you stick to a well-known brand. It is a slightly costlier product, but it is worth its value.

Green Tea Extract

You would have read a lot of articles which correlate green tea with weight loss. These claims are true to an extent. Green tea helps in weight loss by increasing your metabolic rate significantly. Thus, it is advised to drink green tea a few minutes before exercising, to get the best effect.

Omega 3 Fatty Acid

This supplement ingredient helps in improving metabolism. There are a lot of other potential advantages of using this element. When it comes to weight loss, it improves metabolism and also helps in increasing immunity of the body.

Caffeine

Caffeine increases energy and helps to reduce craving for food, at odd times. It suppresses your appetite and thus, you eat less. There are many other benefits of caffeine as well, including stimulating alertness.

There are a lot of elements which are available in supplement form for weight loss like apple cider vinegar and so on. There are some points to consider, before we wind up this chapter.

1. No matter what supplement you choose, diet and exercise are essential for weight loss. Most of the supplements aid in weight loss and do not directly make you lose weight.

2. The brand and quality of supplements are very important factors. Do not buy anything because it is

advertised well or provide offers. Research about the product, learn about advantages and disadvantages and then start using it. If you have any life threatening medical history, it is better to consult a doctor before you consume a supplement.

It is not a crime to use supplements. It can help you gain your target weight as soon as possible. Make sure you consume a lot of water, while you are using these supplements.

Conclusion

Thank you again for downloading this book! I hope it was able to help you start flexible dieting. The next step is to actually start the process. It will not be easy. You will find a lot of hurdles and other problems along the way. Take one step at a time.

If you enjoyed this book, I would really love it if you could give it a review on Amazon.

Happy dieting!